Dedications

This book is dedicated to my mother for making me the person I am, who taught me how to be a good person, how to achieve what I dream, who is a strong and prime example of the person I hope to be like someday and who I have the utmost respect for, she is my idol,

My husband, for being the wonderful man he is, showing me what is really important in life, being by my side through life's trials and listening to all of my frustrations about healthcare throughout the 17 years since we have known each other, he is my rock,

And finally, to my three sons, who spent many days asking when mom would be finished studying and supported me by showing their understanding while I was in nursing school and being my motivation, they will always be my heart.

I love you all...that is what life is about.

CHAPTER ONE
EXPECTATIONS AND HOW IT ALL STARTED

When we are faced with dealing with something we know nothing about, something that can determine whether we live or die, there is a natural feeling of fear and anticipation. In times such as these, it is only instinct to turn somewhere for help. In situations like those we search for someone who has the most possible knowledge that can give us options and guide us through until we can get our lives back to normal. We also turn to family and friends for support, if we have anyone. Ultimately when we are rushed to the hospital because we have chest pain, shortness of breath, severe pain anywhere on our body, if we collapse, if we suddenly have slurred speech and of course, when we have suffered any trauma. At that moment, we place our lives in the hands of the people who have been trained and have become highly skilled to handle these problems, we experience fear and anticipation of what is to come but at that moment we put our TRUST in Physicians and Nurses to help us and to stick to the Hippocratic oath they took to keep us safe and not cause any harm and have our best interest at heart.

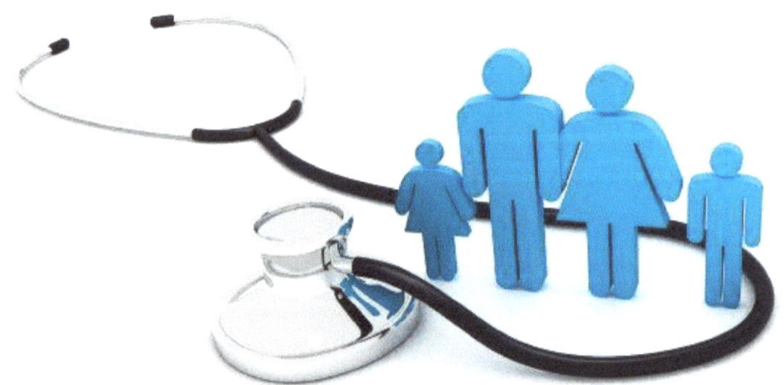

What if I told you that is not what happens, what if I told you some Physicians put their golf game before the birth of your baby and actually tell the nurses to hold you off until they are finished and then they will come. What if I told you that you could actually be in severe pain, visit the emergency room, have diagnostic testing to find out why you are experiencing that pain, be treated for what caused it to "flare up" and make it unbearable, you can actually have diagnostic tests in your record which show a new diagnosis, one for which you can be given options to eradicate and have a long future with your loved ones making new memories, but you happened to have been assigned to a hospitalist who had a date that day or a tee time that afternoon and instead of taking the time to do what any other prudent physician would do, what he took a Hippocratic oath to do and what he initially became a physician to do……he or she just writes discharge orders and decides he doesn't have time to go through the "long, drawn-out, bothersome process" of informing you that you have a new diagnosis of cancer and what that means in terms of what your expectations should be, what your options for treatment are, what if that physician doesn't do a thing but leave that hospital and send you home, only to maybe a few months, maybe a year later, suddenly experience severe pain again, but this time it is much worse, you are rushed to the emergency room, you are assigned a different hospitalist who enters your room and asks you who your oncologist is? If you had chemotherapy or radiation? You are left looking at that doctor like, what are you talking about? Why would I have an Oncologist? Why would I have had chemotherapy or radiation? You must have someone else's record there because I don't have cancer.

Oh, but…..you do have cancer, you have cancer now, you had cancer then when you visited the emergency room months or years prior but no one told you, no one told your family and since no one was informed, you now are being told there is nothing they can do, the cancer has metastasized throughout your body and has spread to your lymph nodes or brain or lungs and is rapidly now taking over your body. You and your family are now devastated….but, you still are unaware that you had it before and no one told you. You just know what you are faced with now and what your family is faced with.

It all sounds like a bad horror movie or nightmare doesn't it? Well it isn't, this happened twice in a period of 14 months to people who went to two different hospitals, two different hospitalists were assigned to these patients but their scenarios were the same. How do I know? I was their home health nurse. I have been a registered nurse for 20 years. I have seen some of the most horrific treatment of other human beings and been completely appalled and horrified that there would be any human being who could do something like that to another human being, a person who was afraid and put their trust in the professional who had been trained and who was supposed to do the right thing...it is sickening and I am disgusted that these situations have taken place. Those poor patients came home, suffered, were discharged by me to hospice services and died within 2 months. They went from living their life day to day without a care to death in 2 months when if they had gotten treatment it is possible their cancer could have been eradicated and they may have gone on to live another 20 or so years, they may not, they may have died in 2 months anyway…..but at least they would have been given a chance and a choice.

Who are they to make that decision for them? They certainly aren't god even though some of them think they are...I have seen physicians look at a patient and think, "oh well, they are 70 years old, they have lived a long life, they will be dying before long anyway, I am not going to do anything for them, it's their time. " No, those words were not said, but if you have been a nurse as long as I have, you know what they are thinking a lot of the time. It is obvious.

Personally, I find that criminal, I find it disgusting and appalling and just have to say, we never know how many years we have left, no matter how old we are. My mother's aunt lived to be 106 years old. Her aunt lived alone and even still drove a car up until the day she died. Her aunt did not suffer in pain, didn't take a pharmacy of medications every day, she lived a wonderful but simple life. Who is to decide someone has lived a long enough life, oh they will just be suffering and dying soon and in pain or whatever the case may be… it isn't some other human being's decision when you have been on this earth long enough now, why bother….sadly something similar to this happened to my mother's sister, her daughters took her to the emergency room, when the people who triaged her asked why she was there, my cousins, not being medical professionals, said "we don't know what is wrong with her but she had some confusion earlier today and some behavior that was not like her and we just are scared she may have had a stroke or something and wanted to bring her in to be sure nothing like that happened…." They took their mother to the emergency room because she had a change in cognition that had never presented before, they were frightened and love their mother with all of their hearts so they rush her to the emergency room for help from people who are supposed to care and who are supposed to do the right thing, the only people who even know how to help you, and they did some diagnostic tests on her, gave her a referral to follow up that week with a urologist, gave her discharge instructions and told her she was free to go. My aunt and my cousins were concerned because no one had mentioned what could be causing both of her legs to become swollen so they asked the doctor to come back in the room and he did, he told her to just follow up with that urologist he told her to see and left the room, my cousins took my aunt home, made her urology appointment the next day for 2 days later and that night found her unresponsive in her bed, called paramedics who came, did CPR and drove her to the hospital where she was put on life support until the next morning when they determined she had no brain waves and was dead. Someone said something to my cousins as to why she died, all in technical terms; they went home to an empty house not understanding what just happened. My cousin decided to call the hospital and try to understand why she was sent home, expressed the concern they had about the swollen legs and were rudely informed that they brought their mother in to find out if she had suffered a stroke, it was ruled out, so she was discharged home, that is what you said when you brought her in and she had not had a stroke so we sent her home……. Wow,……..unbelievable,….. I don't even know what to say about that. The professionals at the hospital asked the untrained loved ones of a patient why they brought her in, ruled that out and without trying to determine why she had a change in cognition and swollen legs just sent her home because it wasn't what they brought her in for… who is supposed to tell who what is wrong with the patient doctor? They didn't care, my aunt was over 80 years old and they decided she lived a long life already; just have her follow up with a urologist in a few days? What if that was their mother, their sister, their daughter, their aunt, their friend, what if that was them? Is that how they would want to be treated? Would that have been acceptable then? We all know the answer to that question. One day that WILL be them. My Mom and aunt's aunt lived to be 106 and have a good quality of life, made lots of memories with her family, how do they know if my aunt could have done the same thing? Unfortunately, my cousins will never know, my patient's families will never know if they could have been able to enjoy more time with their dear loved one. That is not ok.

It was 1993, I was working in the property management business, following in my mother's footsteps, which was a successful business woman and had raised me as a single mother. I had reached the highest position I could achieve in apartment management I was the manager of a 144 unit apartment complex in Henderson, Nevada, my occupancy averaged 92-98% occupied and I didn't feel challenged anymore. I heard about a job where I could work at a casino on the Las Vegas strip and make a lot of money. What I considered a lot of money at the time anyway. The job was primarily dominated by men due to the nature of the job; it was a job as a bellman at the Mirage Hotel and Casino. I decided to apply and I wrote the manager of that department a letter and told him why he should hire me for that position, because of my excellent customer service skills, my bubbly personality and I went on to explain why I was the right person for the job. A little time passed, I wrote him another letter and told him I looked forward to the opportunity to interview for that position. Soon after, the phone rang; it was the assistant of the manager of the Guest Services Department at The Mirage. I couldn't believe it, I was so excited. I went to the interview and was greeted by a man who had a tailored black silk suit on and black dress shoes, not one hair out of place, had a last name you would hear in a movie made about Las Vegas and the old days when the mob ran the town. He was just as full of personality as he was dressed for the part, very friendly and classy, walked with his head held high. We went on a tour of the department and all the other employees looked at me like, oh no, she can't handle this job; this is who you are hiring to work with us? As I walked through there in a fashionable sweater dress and high heels. I had gotten the job, I couldn't believe it, the manager told me he hired me because I was persistent and didn't stop trying. I proceeded to work there and carry my weight as only the second female to ever be hired in that position in the history of The Mirage until I injured my knee, had to have 2 knee surgeries. It was definitely an experience I am glad I had and for a sheltered girl from Texas, I learned a lot about people that I didn't know. So, it was at that time I realized it was time to find a career that would be rewarding, offer a challenge and one where I could make enough money to support myself, as I am a very independent person. I remember looking at the Community College catalog and wondering what I might like to do. I remember trying to decide between court reporting and Nursing, wow, now that

I look back, that was rather odd, two totally different ends of the spectrum. I found myself drawn to the nursing idea, the more I thought about it , the more it was clear to me that it would be the career for me, I would be able to help people in need and make a real difference in people's lives. Let's remember, I had no medical background, no one in my family had any medical background either. I had never worked in that environment as a CNA or anything; I had no clue what it would be like.

Being a single mother of 3 sons at the time, I worked full-time while taking my prerequisite classes; the nursing program was very difficult to get into. There was a waiting list and you were selected by GPA of your pre-requisites, meaning I had to make strait As to even get in. So a 2 year degree, Associates in Applied Science/Nursing, was actually going to take me 4 years, that didn't matter, one thing about me, when I decide to do something, something I really want to do, there is definitely no stopping me. My mother, being an accomplished business woman taught me to think that way. The way I see it, if anyone else in this world can do something, I can do it too. We are no different from each other really, I can be taught to do the same thing anyone else is taught to do and vice-versa.

Fall semester of 1996 came and I began my pre-requisite classes and I got all As and applied for the nursing program and was accepted for the following semester. This, however, presented a little bit of a challenge because now, in the nursing program, there is a schedule you have to follow, you have to attend clinical training every semester in relation to the area of nursing you are learning. Clinicals were every Tuesday and Thursday and they were from 0600 until 1230 and of course, being a single parent, I still had to work to survive and lets not forget studying, and when I say studying, it is learning a whole new language and add in the fact that you had to take a dosage and calculations test and could only miss one question or you were out of the nursing program and had to reapply.

Nursing students report to area hospitals on various floors with their instructor present who then assigns the student to a staff nurse who works at the hospital who then lets you follow them around while you are there and is supposed to offer to let you assist with the skills you are learning at that time and let you help them take care of their patients while you are there. Yeah right, let's be realistic, Nurses do not like student nurses, there is an old saying in nursing and actually, it is quite disgusting, but the saying is, "nurses eat their young." In a perfect world, a student nurse would show up at the hospital and be assigned to a staff nurse who would realize the student is there to help them that day and really can lighten their load a little by answering their call lights, getting supplies they may need, administer medications for at least one of their patient's with their instructor present to be sure they are doing it safely and observing the 4 rights of medication administration; the right patient, right medication , right dose and right time. Reality was, I remember like it was yesterday, I arrived at the county hospital in my 3rd of 4 semesters and my instructor was looking for a nurse to assign me to, she had saved me for last, she could see the nurses were finished with report and were getting ready to start their day so she yelled out, "who would like to take a student today?" the response was about 3 or 4 of the 6 nurses saying "I don't have time for a student, don't give them to me" , "I don't want a student , it slows me down , they are too needy." So, I said "oh ok, no one wants my help, huh, what a shame." Well, needless to say, that day I had to be assigned to a nurse who didn't want to help me and was irritated she had to have a student at all, I learned to be tough and realize that only showed ignorance on their part for not wanting the help I was able to provide and for not wanting to help the new generation of nurses grow into excellent nurses, like some of them had become……let me just point out, it all started there, that was where reality of the industry started to present itself, but I was still thinking positively and I was going to change the world with being the best super nurse anyone had seen , I would show them.

I graduated second in my class in May 2000 and registered for THE EXAM. No, I wasn't a nurse yet; I had to pass my state board exam. It was only a few years that it had been computerized instead of paper and the deal was you could get anywhere between 75 and 265 questions on your exam, depending on how you answered each question. It was a test to pull your general knowledge of nursing out if you had it. There was a rumor that if you only got 75 questions, you passed for sure, if you got more than that, it wasn't sure and you would just have to wait the 6 weeks it took to receive your results in the mail. That is so cruel, 6 weeks. It seems like 6 months. Well, I took the exam and only got 75 questions but that test is so hard that it doesn't matter; everyone comes out of there thinking they failed, and there was not one person who said they felt extremely confident coming out of there. You take it at a testing center and you usually aren't there with anyone you know, and it takes as long as 5-6 hours to take the test. I had taken a preparation course for the exam and I still felt like I didn't pass, but I did. Six weeks later I received notice that I passed, and I was actually a registered nurse finally after 4 years.

Next, was getting a job that hired new grads, most hospitals and most specialty areas have new grad programs where you have an eight- week course and are assigned to a preceptor before you are on your own. I decided to go into Labor and Delivery, I got the job and was assigned to a preceptor on the unit, everyone from the class was looking for their preceptors on the floor to meet them and I watched as some of my class mates met theirs and I was then looking for my preceptor, I asked someone, who is Theresa? They said, "Oh, you got Captain Rhodes?" I said "yes, what do you mean captain?" They said, "your preceptor is a former Army captain" I gasped, "oh dear god, help me Jesus" and soon I met captain Rhodes, she was intimidating, she was very professional, very calm, direct and spoke softly but with firm demeanor. I didn't know how to feel or what to think at first and I remember thinking, wow, it doesn't matter what question these patients ask her, she knows the answer to all of them and doesn't have to say let me find out for you, I was in awe, she knew all and I remember thinking I hope one day I will be able to answer everyone's questions as easily as she can, that was my goal, to be able to do that and do it as eloquently as she did.

One day I reported to captain Rhodes and it was time for me to start my first IV, I figured she would tell me to start it on one of our patients, no...I was to start it on her, I broke out in an instant waterfall, forget sweat, I was drenched and couldn't breathe, felt like I would pass out and was terrified!!! What if I didn't get it, what if I hurt her somehow, other than the normal pain of having an 18gauge needle shoved in your veins...I wanted to go hide under a desk or something but knew it was something I had to do and I had to get myself together and not let her know how scared I was. So, I went to get the supplies and proceeded to prepare to start the IV. Thank goodness I did it, it went like clock-work, I had just gotten lucky by the grace of god but I had successfully started my first IV on my preceptor, Army captain Rhodes x 1 attempt. I was on cloud 10 and stayed there the rest of the day. I soon realized I was glad to be assigned to captain Rhodes, she did things right and she made sure I knew why I was doing what I was doing so I really learned everything the right way and I went on to have the confidence to work as an agency nurse who is then expected to function in a work environment where I had never been but function like I had been part of the team for years and I chose to challenge myself to learn so many areas of nursing and experience so many wonderful learning opportunities, one of the facilities I worked for as an agency nurse agreed to buy out my contract with the agency I worked for and hire me on full-time. Actually, that happened several times while I worked agency. As a result of all of those experiences I was recognized by Nathan Adelson Hospice, Las Vegas Chamber of Commerce, The March of Dimes, Healthsouth Desert Canyon Rehabilitation Hospital, Valley Hospital Medical Center, Universal Home Health, The World Nursing Congress and Women of Distinction, the Honors Version. I was fortunate to have the learning experiences I had and unfortunately that lead to me seeing just how corrupt and wrong this profession, just like so many others, really is.

There was actually one occasion where the doctor had forgotten to write an order for potassium for a patient I was taking care of one day on a med-surg floor and the patient was going to be discharged home that day and I went in to her room, took her vital signs, left her room and continued to take the rest of my patient's vital signs and was down the hallway by then when the doctor went in the room and the patient was unresponsive and he yelled for me to come help, I ran down and my patient was blue, I called a code and the code team came up and tried to save my patient but was unable. My patient wasn't very old, maybe in her early 50s and she was discharging home that morning, but when that happened the doctor had tried to take the chart and I heard him saying, I know I ordered potassium yesterday, but the truth was, he hadn't and he was trying to put the order in the chart and then blame nursing for not following his orders. When I heard him say that I went and grabbed the chart from him and did not give it back to him until the house supervisor was there so she could see that there was no order for potassium in the chart. After she came up and I showed her that there was no order for potassium I went down to the main floor, busted outside and cried and cried that my patient was dead and I remember calling my mother and crying to her that I was sad because my patient had died and it wasn't right, she should be alive and have gotten to go home. That was a rough shift, I will never forget it, and I soon quit working at that hospital and went into a different area of nursing after that.

Call me naive, I just always had been taught, doctors do what is right and they help people. I guess I had lived a little bit of a sheltered life but the things I have seen since becoming a nurse have really opened my eyes to a different world, where doctors are not only trying to blame others for their malpractice but they are doing surgeries that are not motivated by necessity, they are motivated by the all mighty dollar. I don't just mean orthopedic surgeries like knee replacements, shoulder replacements, I am talking about neurosurgeries, brain surgeries, back surgeries and abdominal surgeries that are unnecessary because they want to make money, they know how to document to make it look necessary, they know exactly what to say in their documentation for it to support the need for the procedures, who is going to question them with all the appropriate documentation? Some procedures it would be impossible to do that with due to needing diagnostic tests prior to performing the procedure that would show it to not be necessary but not all. It is actually pretty frightening. There are many surgeries on the back and many orthopedic elective surgeries that should never happen. People put trust in the surgeons and think if they are suggesting it, then it must be necessary, that is because they trust the doctors to do the right thing. I am going to now give you some advice that I have come to see is necessary to keep you safe and hopefully decrease the likelihood of something horrific happening to you. So let's get to the whole point of this, let's get to what has motivated me to write this in the first place, that is to tell you how to keep you and your loved ones from being victim and if something I recommend can save at least one life, then this will not be in vein.

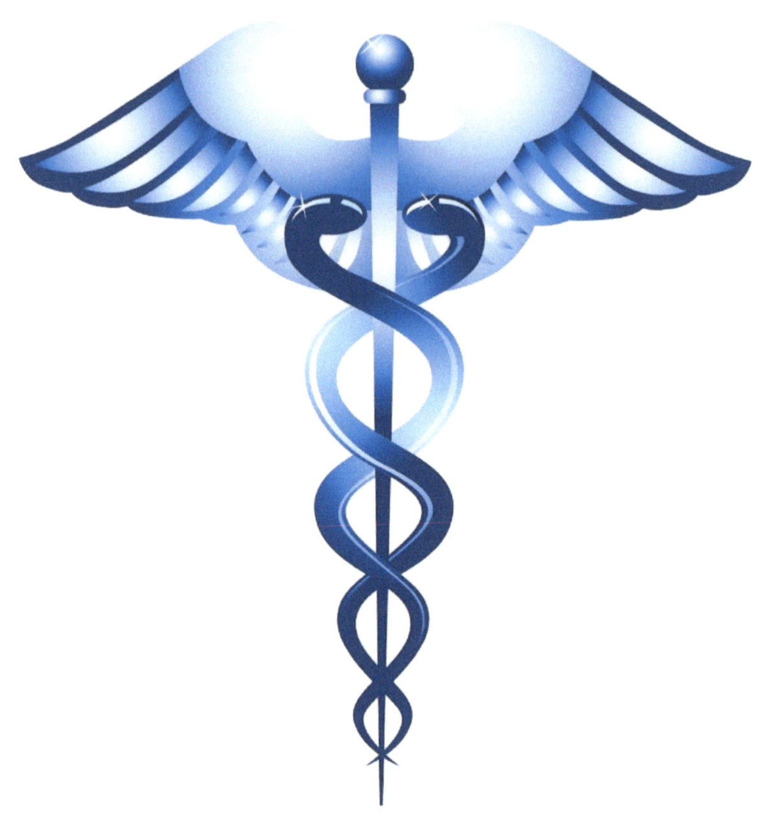

Prior to the Covid-19 virus, it was ok to stay with your loved one in their room and not leave them alone to have no attention when they may need it or whatever the circumstance, at least there could be someone present watching over them to be sure they weren't treated poorly. We will have to see what happens as a result of the Covid-19 situation but if things change back to how they were before this at least to the point of letting family members be with the patient while they are in the hospital, then that is what needs to happen, do not EVER leave a loved one in the hospital alone, ever. Someone should be there 24/7 from the time they go to the emergency room until the day they are discharged and there should be two family members taking turns, one sleeps and showers at home while the other stays with the patient and they can relieve each other. This is very important, this will prevent staff members from being rude or mean to the patient, from forgetting to reconnect their oxygen after they return to the room after being taken down to get x-rays, CT scans or whatever they may have needed to be taken from their room for. Be sure the person who is with the patient is aware of all of the tests the patient is due to have and each time the doctor comes in to see the patient , make sure the person who is there with the patient asks questions about what the doctor will be ordering and why. It is your right as the patient to know what tests the doctor is ordering and why. Be sure to ask every doctor who interacts with the patient that question and it doesn't matter if the doctor seems irritated at that or not, it is your right. Do it, it may save your life, be sure the doctor can explain the reason he is ordering the test also.

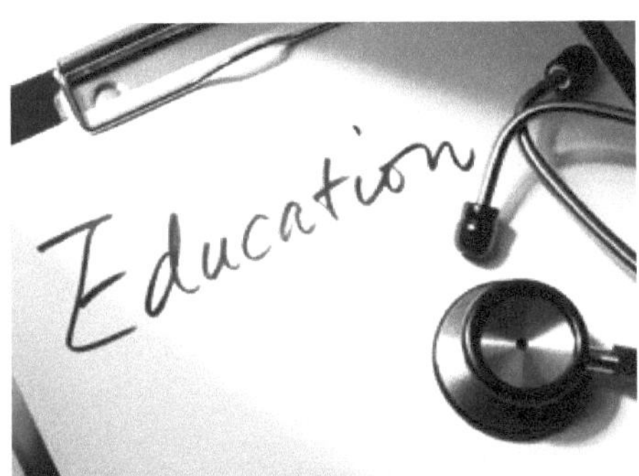

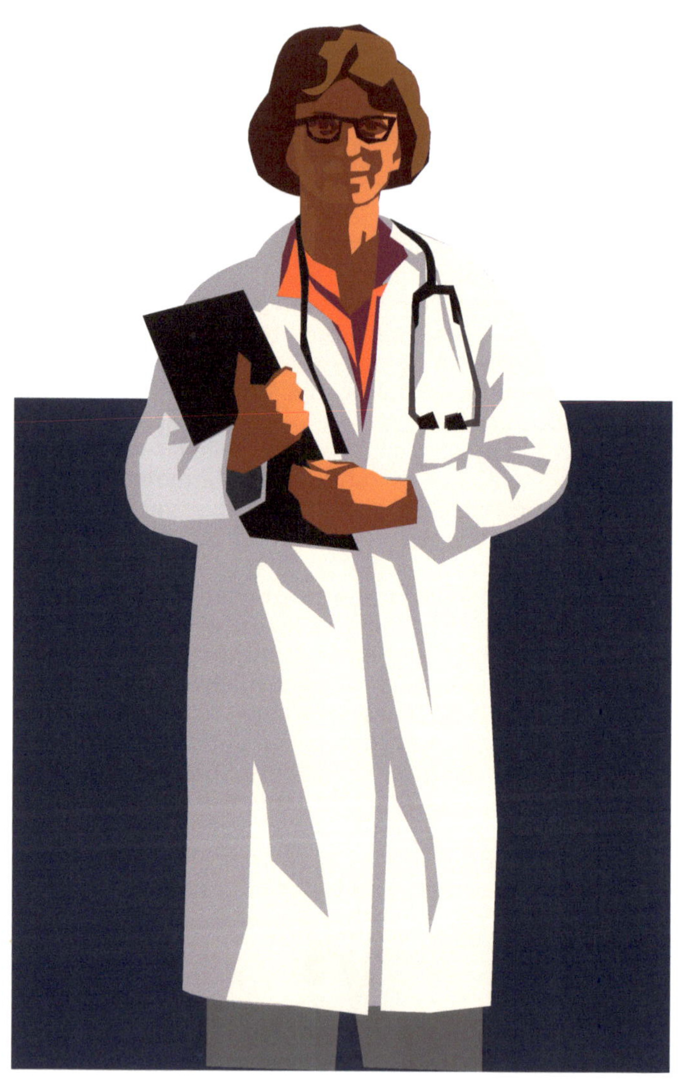

CHAPTER THREE

ASK EVERY NURSE WHO GIVES MEDICATION WHAT THEY ARE GIVING.

I know we would all like to think when someone is entering our hospital room to give us medicine, we should just be able to trust that it is the correct medicine and we should just take it because the doctor and the nurse said so…WRONG! Please, do not do that. Please remember several things that are very important to remember in that situation; doctors and nurses are human and unfortunately, they make mistakes. I will speak for myself as a nurse when I say I am not perfect by any means, but I have never made a medication error in my 20-year career as a nurse, thank god.

It is every patient's right to know what the nurse is giving them, it doesn't matter if it is a pill, injection or an IV medication, every patient should be informed of what they are given, EVERY TIME. What most people don't know is there are five rights to be considered when nurses are passing medication, they are all taught this in nursing school and I guarantee when they are passing medication in the hospital with their instructor present when they are just nursing students, their instructor is closely watching to see if the nurse is mindful of the five rights. The five rights are right patient, right medication, right dose, right time and right route. The nurse should always check the armband of the patient prior to administering medication of any type to the patient to be sure it is the right patient, the nurse is always supposed to open the medication in front of the patient and tell the patient the name and dosage of the medication they are opening, the nurse should always check the physician's order carefully to be sure of the route the medication is to be given since there are some medications that can be given by mouth, by injection and by IV, the nurse is also supposed to be sure the medication is given within the hour of when it is scheduled.

Now, just think about what I just said, the medication is to be given to the patient within an hour, no later, of when it is scheduled, so, if the nurse is working in an acute hospital, she or he may be assigned anywhere between 6 and 10 patients each. The nurse is responsible for passing medication to all of those patients and usually when a patient is in the hospital, they have no fewer than 10-23 medications to take and sometimes those medications are to be taken more than once a day. Most medications are due in the morning; all of your daily medication is typically given in the morning at 0800-0900. If you have any medication that is taken three times a day, it will be given 1100-1200 usually, then again at 2200 with the nighttime medication. Diabetics also have to have their blood sugar checked prior to being given insulin, when diabetic patients are in the hospital; their blood sugar is checked 4 times per day. Another thing to realize if you are diabetic, when you are a patient in the hospital, a lot of times, even when you don't take insulin at home, normally, you will be given insulin at the hospital. The reason you are given insulin in the hospital is because when a diabetic is sick enough to be admitted to the hospital, their body is under extra stress and when that happens, your blood sugar will be higher. Most of the time the physician will order a sliding scale for your insulin, meaning; the amount of insulin you are given is going to depend on your blood glucose level. Sliding scales usually begin if blood sugar results are above 150. If your blood sugar is 150-155, you may get 2 units of regular insulin, and then if 156-200, you may get 4 units of regular insulin and so on until if your blood sugar is 400 or higher, you may get 12-14 units of regular insulin and the nurse is to call the doctor for further orders. Also, if you are diabetic, you are to be given a snack at 2200 just before bed.

Now, we have to also realize that every patient has what is called PRN medication, PRN medication is medication that is to be given to the patient as needed. There are several points to remember about PRN medication; the doctor may write an order that basically says give the patient a certain pain medication every 4 hours as needed and the doctor will indicate the route but what people don't understand about as needed medication is the patient is to be given that medication only if they ask for it or complain of a symptom that the medication order is written for by the doctor. A typical order for pain medication may be written as follows: Percocet 5/500mg 1-2 tablets q 6 hrs prn pain. That means to give the patient 1 or 2 tablets of Percocet 5/500mg every 6 hours as needed for pain, meaning if the patient states they are having pain.

If a nurse has several diabetic patients with sliding scale insulin along with their other ordered medications, which as we just discussed, may be several times a day, and if the patient has prn medication, which all patients have ordered, you can imagine, the nurse pretty much spends her entire shift passing medication to her patients and documenting her assessment, which is something a registered nurse is required to do every shift in an acute care hospital.

My point with all of that is...that leaves a lot of room for error. The nurse should always ask the patient when she brings a patient a prn medication because the CNA reported to him or her that the patient asked for something to help them sleep or the patient pushed the call button for pain medicine, or whatever the need is, the nurse should still ask the patient when they enter the room if the patient requested any medication for whatever the CNA reported to them, just always remember, no human being is perfect and the CNA may have told the nurse the wrong patient...there are so many things that can go wrong and cause a medication error.

Sometimes there may be nurses who think they know everything and become too relaxed about giving medication and that is the dangerous nurse, not the student, who has her instructor watching her, but the nurse who thinks they know everything and who gets in a hurry and who skips being mindful of the five rights of medication administration.

Please just always keep those things in mind. Clinicians have access to approximately 10,000 medications. Each year medication errors account for 700,000 ER visits and 100,000 Hospitalizations, also 5% of hospitalized patients are given wrong medications and experience adverse drug reactions, meaning, it causes the patient harm. Every year 7000 – 9000 people die from being given the wrong medication in the hospital. Another horrible reality is medical errors are the third leading cause of death in the United States. Yes, I said the **third** leading cause of death. That is extremely alarming. Now do you think you may need to finish reading this book?

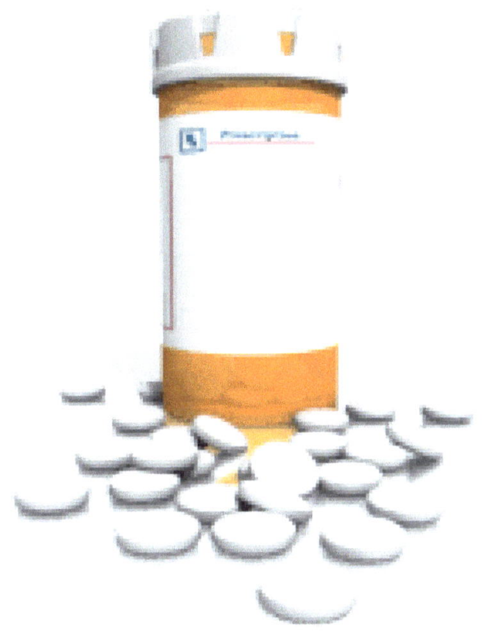

CHAPTER FOUR
PAIN MANAGEMENT

While we are on the subject of medication, let's also discuss pain management. I won't get stuck on my soap box about this because I could go on for days about how wrong it is that nurses do not appropriately administer pain medication to patients and make them suffer. I will never forget how appalling it is to go to work as a nurse in a hospital and receive report from the off going nurse who describes any patient as "drug seeking". Let me just put it this way, I can't remember a time I received report from a nurse who didn't describe a patient as drug seeking. I don't know what happened to people in the medical profession that made them forget people really do experience pain. THEY REALLY DO EXPERIENCE PAIN. I swear, it is so frustrating to me. I must tell you about a couple of experiences I had in the acute care hospital that blow my mind.

One time I was working as an agency nurse and reported to a local hospital on the medical-surgical floor and as soon as I got off of the elevator of the unit I was to report to I heard a man yelling profanity and just carrying on with every other word being the "F" word. I was working the night shift that night and it is a well-known fact, as I mentioned already, that agency nurses get the most difficult patients so the staff nurses don't have to bother with them and can spend their extra time gossiping or whatever they wanted to do besides work. Anyway, I knew the upset gentleman would be my patient that night and I was right. It was explained to me in report that the patient was a prisoner and was a self-proclaimed heroin addict but that he was in the hospital because he had fractured his femur. Hmmm, let's see…last I knew, a fractured bone was pretty darn painful and a fractured femur requires surgery and is considered a medical emergency, the fact that there is a fracture as a diagnosis also means there has been an X-ray to confirm the bone is actually broken, so there is no way there could be any confusion regarding whether there is a fracture or not. During the report the nurse said to me that the patient was "drug seeking" that always refers to pain medication, meaning the patient is just a drug addict wanting pain medication.

When a nurse arrives to start his or her shift, the first thing they should do, after receiving report, is go to each patient and introduce themselves and make sure their patient is alive and ok. I would always make this the first thing I did when I arrived to let the patient know who I am and that I would be returning shortly to do their assessment and administer their medication. I also took that opportunity to check with the patients to see if they needed pain medication if it was due or if their prn medication was able to be administered yet. I learned long ago, if you make your patients comfortable and take care of their needs at the beginning of the shift, your call lights will not be going off all night long and your patients will get better rest at night, allowing them to feel better the next day.

Anyway, I went in to my upset patient's room to introduce myself and he was furious and cursing and I knew why, I explained to him I would return with pain medication for him and that I would then pass my medications and then as soon as I was finished with that, I would bring his chart into his room and we could work out a schedule for his pain medication to help relieve his pain since he had not only 1 but 2 different IV pain medications ordered and 1 by mouth break through pain medication ordered by the physician. He said "yeah, whatever, f ***, you probably won't be back the rest of the night." I assured him I would be right back with his pain med and then return so we could discuss our plan. I immediately came back and gave him one of his IV pain medications, I gave him his scheduled medication at the same time and then went to see my other patients and administer their scheduled medications, I then returned to my upset patient's room , as I had promised to do, and brought his chart and we discussed our plan, basically, I told him what I thought would work best for him and what all he had ordered and I also told him I could see that he had not been given any of his ordered pain medication and that I was sure he must be in excruciating pain and I apologized that none of the other nurses had helped him. Between the IV medication he had ordered and the by mouth pain medication and the sleep aid he had ordered, I was hoping to be able to relieve his pain enough that he could rest comfortably. I considered it part of my responsibility as a nurse to help this poor man not suffer.

The main problem with the whole situation is; the man had pain medication ordered by the physician, let's think about this really well...**ordered by the physician,** there is usually a very good reason medication is ordered by a physician...wouldn't you imagine? It doesn't take a nurse to understand that. The poor man had this pain medication ordered and the day shift nurse did not give him any. You can't tell me she didn't know he needed it, the whole hospital probably knew he needed it, he was yelling loudly throughout report when I arrived at the unit. I immediately knew he needed it. What was she, stupid? No, well, yeah, but that is a whole other ball of wax. Let's just tell it like it is, she is one of the majority of nurses out there, unfortunately, most nurses consider patients to be drug seeking if they ask for pain medication. Guess what? Even if the patient is "drug seeking", I don't care. That's right, I said, I don't care. Let me explain why; in nursing school you are taught the only way to know if anyone is in pain is if they say they are in pain and the only way to know the magnitude of the patient's pain is by listening to the patient when they explain their pain. It is that simple!!!!!! Pain cannot be measured; there is no diagnostic test to tell a clinician how much pain someone is experiencing. There is no way to know if a person is in pain or how much pain they are in besides listening to the patient explain that to you.

I once took my adult son to the emergency room because he reported vomiting black coffee ground emesis. That is indicative of a stomach ulcer. I took him to the emergency room to get help for him and his younger brother happened to be visiting and had decided to go with us. We entered the emergency room, signed in and took a seat. On the sign in sheet, you are to state why you are there so you can be called in a priority of severity of complaint. We sat a few minutes and my son was called to triage, he was triaged and then returned to the emergency room waiting room with my youngest son and me. We waited for an extended period of time for him to be called back to be seen, during that wait, my sons were talking and catching up with each other and making jokes and carrying on and it should be noted, my son who was being seen in the emergency room is quite the jokester with a very funny sense of humor and he and his brother were carrying on having a good ole time. My son was finally called in to see the doctor and went through some diagnostic tests and when he was finished came out to check out and explained to me and his brother that he had 2 stomach ulcers and the physician had written him approximately 4 prescriptions, two that he was going to need to take regularly every day from now on. He told us that one of the ulcers was perforated. I don't know if you know much about perforated stomach ulcers, but they are very painful. Stomach acid leaks out of the stomach into places it doesn't belong and that hurts very much. My son obviously has a very high pain tolerance and even though he was in pain, he was sitting in the waiting room of the emergency room laughing with his brother right before being diagnosed with a perforated stomach ulcer. Do you get what I am saying here…obviously you cannot go by how a patient looks, their behavior, whether they are sleeping or anything you see because they can still be in a lot of pain. People deal with pain differently and it is wrong to assume you know someone is not in pain or how much pain they are in.

Back to my poor patient, I followed the plan we had decided on, exactly as we had discussed together. Pretty soon, there was no yelling occurring, no profanity, no disruptive behavior, I checked on him throughout the evening and when the dayshift nurse returned, she could not believe that the patient was sleeping and not yelling or cursing. I reported off and left the hospital.   That day, the staffing agency I worked for called me and told me that hospital was requesting me to return to the same unit and asked me if I could work, I said yes and went back, I was assigned the same patients with the exception of the ones who had been discharged home already and went in to see them all at the beginning of the shift as I always did and the upset patient from the night before greeted me very kindly and said, "oh, I am so glad you are back, I didn't get to see you before you left this morning, I wanted to thank you so much for helping me, last night was the first night I slept since I broke my femur and I wanted to thank you so much for relieving my pain so I actually got to sleep." I replied, "Yes, sir, I am happy to help you and if that was me in that bed with a broken femur, I would want someone to help me too." I smiled and told him I would be right back with his pain medicine and we would follow our same plan as we did the night before. He was happy and there was no yelling and he had another night of rest and all I did was follow doctor's orders and help him figure out a plan to make those orders work for him so he didn't have to suffer.

The other incident that stands out in my mind, when it comes to pain, is much more brief, but just as profound; I was working on a medical-surgical floor of a local hospital, which I worked at often, as an agency nurse. I had a patient who had not been compliant with going to dialysis and her port had gone bad, meaning she could not receive dialysis through it anymore. The doctor who was to replace the catheter came in and since it was my patient and I was responsible to assist him, I washed up and put on all my garb for the sterile procedure and went in the room, the doctor was there and ready to begin the procedure, the patient had a drape over her head and the new catheter was going to be placed in her neck. My patient was somewhat afraid and since the physician had arrived at the hospital without any warning, the patient had not been given anything for anxiety or pain prior to this procedure. I assisted the physician in preparing for the procedure while maintaining sterility and then offered my had to the patient, who was terrified, the physician, who did nothing to make my patient comfortable, began to make an incision on my patient's neck to insert the huge catheter through, my patient screamed, I told her she could squeeze my hand as hard as she needed to and she did, I stared at the physician and when he looked up at me after torturing my patient by shoving that huge catheter through the incision he made, while my patient screamed and pled for mercy, there is no doubt he could see the disgust I had for him through my tear-filled eyes. I was so angry and had such compassion for my patient and at the time such disgust and disbelief for that physician, I had begun to cry, out of pure anger. I glared straight through him and didn't say one word other than telling my patient I was there for her and she could squeeze my hand as hard as she wanted to.   I am a nurse, I know patients have to experience pain sometimes and there is nothing we can do about that, but give me a break, there is **NO** reason that patient should not have been able to be medicated prior to the procedure, even if the physician would have at least injected some lidocaine, or anything first, that would have been more acceptable, but the doctor did not care! He could have cared less, he saw a non-compliant patient, blamed her for her port not working anymore and decided to "teach her a lesson", that was obvious. I NEVER FORGOT THE HORROR OF THAT.

Needless to say, I continued my career and always kept my pledge to help my patients and do anything I could to keep them as comfortable, as possible, in their time of need while they were my patient. I was frequently outraged at the lack of concern for patients in the healthcare industry. I just believe we should do unto others as we would have them do unto us. It is really the only thing that is right in my mind. I often look at the world and think, what has happened to everyone? What happened to society and why are they all so desensitized? It is terrible, I find myself thinking that in many different situations that actually have nothing to do with healthcare also, but that is another ball of wax that I am not talking about in this book. But it is clear, something has got to change!

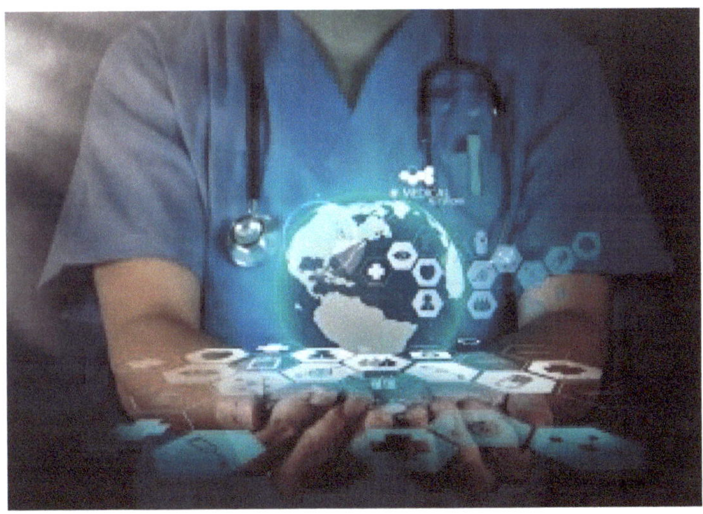

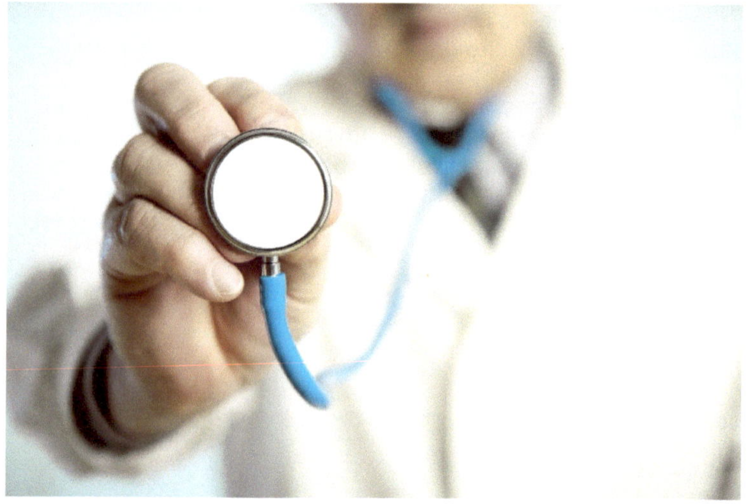

Now, let's discuss physicians, wow, where do I begin, I will make this short but to the point, the first thing you should know is…you have a right, as a patient in the hospital, or any other situation actually, to fire your physician. A lot of people do not know that. Please, whatever you do, remember, that physician would not even have a job if it were not for patients, would they? That is something they tend to forget sooooooo frequently.

If a physician is a hospitalist working in the community, they are frequently privileged to work in many of the surrounding hospitals and they are assigned patients when they are in the on-call rotation for that particular hospital. For instance, let's say you go to the emergency room for abdominal pain. You see the emergency room doctor, he decides you need to be admitted to the hospital for monitoring or for further diagnostic testing to determine what is wrong with you since you are not stable enough to go home and make an appointment with a specialist or your primary care physician to order testing, or you may need emergency surgery or blood thinners due to having a stroke or whatever the case may be, you are then assigned an internal medicine doctor, who is your main doctor throughout your hospitalization, the doctor who will order consults with specialist physicians who will then visit you, do their own assessments, order their own tests, and give the internal medicine physician their report of their findings. If they believe you need immediate attention, they inform the internal medicine doctor and arrangements begin to accommodate their request.

This information is vital because if you, as the patient, do not speak up and request more information, the ball will keep rolling and you will then be presented with a document called an informed consent...ok, informed means informed, last I checked anyway. So, the informed consent is usually a document that is pre-printed and has a blank where the name of the procedure is filled in. The informed consent is a document that is required to be signed by the patient or patient's legal representative, prior to any procedure being done on a patient in any hospital, in the United States, unless it is a life-saving procedure that you are unconscious for and have no legal representative present. That is the only exception to that rule. If the patient has a DNR classification, meaning the patient desires no life saving techniques be used, should they go into cardiac arrest, then the staff is to only stand by and allow the person to pass on. If there is uncertainty as to the patient's classification, such as in a trauma unit and no one knows what the patient's desires are, everything will be done to save the patient's life.

Ok, back to speaking up regarding what is going on in the hospital, you are there, you have been assigned an internal medicine physician to manage your case while you are admitted to an acute care hospital, the only thing you know is a bunch of different doctors come in and ask you the same questions over and over and the lab people seem like you are the never ending source for Dracula's nutrition, they come in at 0300 or 0400 or whatever time it may be, but it is always early in the morning, when you are just getting to sleep, and they turn on the brightest light ever created and put a tourniquet around your arm that makes you feel like they are going to amputate it right then and there then they take like 6 tubes of blood, AGAIN, and leave the room. The doctor, who is your internal medicine doctor, who is required to round on you (see you) everyday, then comes in as soon as you fall back asleep and puts his stethoscope on your chest and listens for 2 seconds, leaves the room and you are so out of it due to lack of sleep you don't even remember him or her visiting you that morning, which means you didn't get any information from him or her at all. Things just keep happening and the next thing you know, an informed consent form is stuck in your face and the nurse tells you that it is an informed consent form for you to have the procedure your physician discussed with you and you look at your nurse like; WHAT?????

If you don't know any better, you may just sign it and the
next thing you know, you don't get anything to eat, all you
can have to put in your mouth at that point is ice chips and
then that is taken away and the next thing you know you
have a whole bunch of people with funny looking hats on
come to get you again while you are trying to sleep and then
you get taken into a very bright, very cold room, with all
kinds of complicated looking equipment, there is a person
with the same type of outfit on that tells you he will make
you comfortable and you can go back to sleep now and the
next thing you know, you wake up wondering why you are
feeling so much pain. This can really happen to you.

The moral of the story is... as a patient anytime, anywhere,
you have the right to ask questions!!! You have to ask
questions because those people, who call themselves
physicians, sadly enough, a lot of times, will not do their job
and inform you of what is going on. It is their job to do that.
Nurses are not supposed to. Your physician, who comes into
your room for anywhere between 3-10 minutes a day, is
supposed to discuss with you what is going on with YOUR
body and what your choices are to do about it and what the
implications are if you do not do what they are suggesting
you do. It is just that simple. The nurse is not the person
who is responsible to tell you that. The nurse is responsible
to obtain informed consent and have you sign that document
only **AFTER** the doctor has informed you of what needs to
happen and you have asked the doctor all of the questions
you wish to ask. That is how it is, cut and dry, pure and
simple, period.

Do not **EVER** let a doctor come in your room and leave
without you being satisfied that you understand everything
they are telling you and why they are suggesting whatever
they are suggesting and what will possibly happen if you do
not do what they are suggesting and what the risks are if
you do what they are suggesting. This is so important. If a
physician ever does this to you, you call for the nurse or
anyone who will listen and you tell them you want to talk to
that doctor who just came to see you and left before you
could even speak. If that doctor does not come right back
in, unless they have left the hospital and then they should
call you on the phone at a minimum, you tell your nurse you
want a different doctor and you don't want that doctor to
come back in your room ever again. You are the boss. It is
your body they are doing things to. Do not let a doctor
come in there and end up sending you a bill for an
outrageous amount of money for not even doing his job
because a part, to me the most important part, of their job
is to keep their patient informed of what is happening to
them.

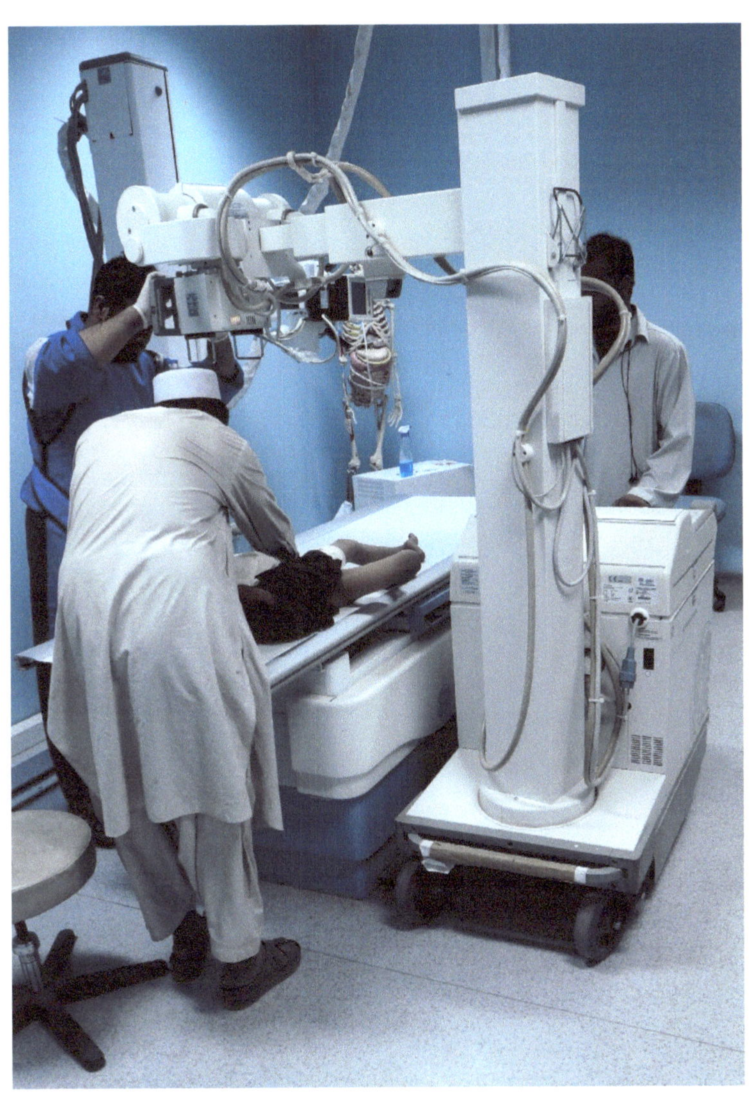

CHAPTER SIX
GET A SECOND OPINION

Do not ever feel worried about questioning your doctor when it comes to their recommendation about treatment. Remember, we already established, you are the boss. Always remember that! It may sound elementary and it kind of is but the way I deal with anything in my life since I became more aware of things and how things are done, I think of this old elementary school saying; "you aren't the boss of me." I actually laugh when I think about it but I do think about it in serious situations also. I mean, it may be elementary, and I graduated from college with honors but there is something to be said for that saying. I use it in how I deal with my life very often.

If your doctor, in a regular walk-in visit with your primary care physician or in the hospital with some internal medicine hospitalist you have never seen before or a specialist in the hospital you have never seen before or anytime you are face to face with any doctor, let's just put it that way, tells you that you need to have a test or a procedure or anything they say that comes out of their mouth, you question them until you understand what they are saying first, then if it is something you feel uncertain about, tell them you want a second opinion. Let's face it, it is your body and the other important point is, if they are a good physician and know what they are doing, they are not going to care about you wanting a second opinion because if they are doing what they are supposed to, the second opinion will recommend the same treatment.

Always be leery and run as fast as you can from anyone who seems bothered by you asking for a second opinion. I don't care what it is about, if they are telling you the truth about what you need done, they will be fine with it because the second opinion will say the same thing they are. It doesn't matter where you are, if you are in the doctor's office, the hospital, on the operating table before you are put to sleep, if you are not sure about what is happening and why and if it is a good idea... DON'T DO IT UNTIL ALL OF YOUR QUESTIONS ARE ANSWERED and you are comfortable with your decision. Notice I said YOUR decision. It is your body and you are the one who has to live with the decision, no one else. Don't let a physician bully you into doing anything or hurrying to do anything. Too bad if he or she is in a hurry, if that is the case, you don't want that doctor anyway.

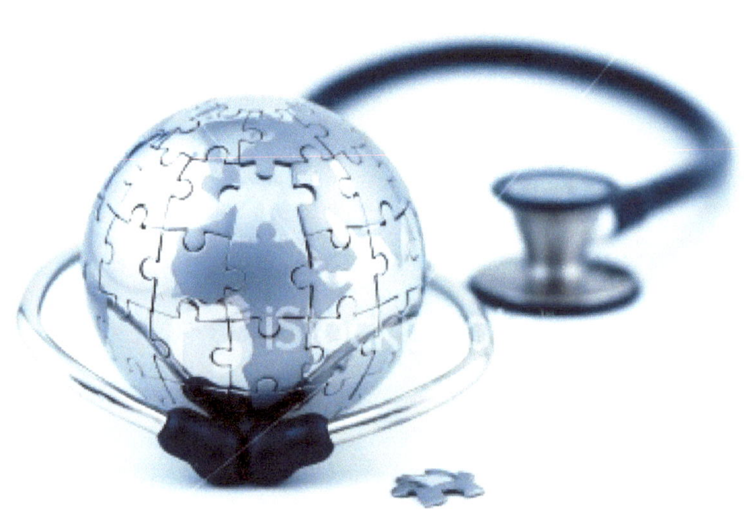

CHAPTER SEVEN
READINESS FOR DISCHARGE

Something everyone needs to know is, there are an estimated number of days a person spends in acute care hospitals. If a person is not then ready for discharge, meaning, safe to go home, then they are typically referred to Skilled Nursing Facilities. These facilities are considered sub-acute care facilities. There are also average lengths of stay in a skilled nursing facility, if a person is not yet ready to discharge home safely from the skilled nursing facility after the average length of stay there the next place is usually a long-term care facility. There are actually a lot of different places for a person to go other than home from the acute care hospital. I will break it down with just a general scenario that might occur.

A person is usually admitted to an acute care hospital from the emergency room. Of course, it depends on why they are admitted and what needs to happen to stabilize the patient's condition as far as how long they may need to be there. If a person is admitted with abdominal pain, they have diagnostic tests done, maybe it is determined they need surgery and if so, that will likely occur the next day, unless it is an absolute emergency; such as appendicitis or a bowel obstruction, anything life threatening will require immediate surgery. Let's say it is not life threatening but must be done before a person would be able to return home, they may have surgery the next morning after admission and then remain in the acute care hospital approximately 2 days. If the patient is stable and everything is going as planned and the patient has no other health conditions, they will be discharged home as long as they will be considered safe to do so...ok that would definitely be an area where I see that happening way too often without the case manager, who is a registered nurse or social worker, doing their job correctly. The case manager in the hospital is responsible to be sure every patient is discharged safely; it is their actual responsibility legally. Let's say a patient has had the surgery and they also are 70 years old and have congestive heart failure, which can make it very difficult to breathe, especially if the person engages in activity, sometimes even as minor as walking. So, if that person is supposed to leave the acute care hospital because they no longer require that level of care but they don't have any family or anyone else to help them at least be sure they get to the bathroom ok for the first few days at home, that patient should not go home and should be referred to a skilled nursing facility.

A skilled nursing facility is staffed with Registered Nurses, Licensed Practical Nurses or some states call them Licensed Vocational Nurses, Certified Nursing Assistants, Physical Therapy teams and Occupational therapy teams (both of which have assistants). The focus in a skilled nursing facility will be to strengthen the patient and get them safe to return home, sometimes they are able to do that in the expected length of stay and sometimes they are not. In the case of the 70 year old patient with congestive heart failure, they would likely be able to get the patient strong enough and train the patient to use assistive devices; walkers, wheelchairs, canes, grabbers, shower chairs, grab bars, raised toilet seats, bedside commodes and rollators, those type of assistive devices , which will help the patient be safe to return home, either with family or caregiver assistance for a while or alone, depending on what happened to cause the patient to go into the hospital in the first place. The average length of stay in a skilled nursing facility can be as long as 60 days. Most of the time, that would be in cases where someone suffered a stroke and their lives have changed drastically because they can no longer do things they used to do and it may take a long time to teach them and their caregiver, if they have one, how to adjust to where the patient is able to be discharged home safely.

Sometimes a patient will just not be able to safely go home anymore. If a patient lives alone and has had a stroke and they have no family to help them and cannot afford the $22.00 per hour to have a Personal Care Attendant 24 hours a day that it may take if the person is severely disabled after the stroke then they would have to be discharged to a long-term care facility. That type of facility is what is known as a nursing home.

I have to take this opportunity to express my feelings on nursing homes. This is just my opinion, but do not forget that I have 20 years of experience as a Registered Nurse and I have worked as an agency nurse in many different facilities, many different levels of care and I will explain to you now how I feel about nursing homes. I am not saying they are all exactly the same, because they are not. There are some very beautiful new nursing homes that are terrible and there are some very old ugly nursing homes that are better than terrible. NONE ARE ACCEPTABLE TO ME. I am sorry, I really feel if I ever get to the point I am not able to take care of myself and none of my children wish to assist me and something happened to my wonderful husband, god forbid and I didn't know anyone who would help and I could not afford help at home, I would prefer to leave the skilled nursing facility against medical advice and take my chances if I was able to even crawl out of there. I would do anything to avoid having to be a patient in any nursing home.

I feel very strongly about that. I have seen nurses be very mean to patients and of course I have reported them. I have started a shift and gone into a paraplegic patient's room and they reek of urine and bowel movement. I have found patients who, it was obvious, had been sitting in a dirty diaper for hours and hours before I got there and let's face it, there is no way every paralyzed patient gets turned off of their bony prominences every 2 hours, which is protocol to prevent pressure ulcers. Sometimes these poor patients have food all over them because some idiot staff member did not help them eat, the patients often have feces under their fingernails and all over them and their wheelchair. It is inhumane the way people are treated in these places.

I mentioned before that it doesn't matter how beautiful and new the building may look, if there are terrible staff members working there, it can be hell. I have absolutely seen patients better cared for and happier at some old ugly nursing homes before.

I remember when I was a nursing student; your first rotation in the clinical setting is a nursing home. You are to assist the staff in caring for the patients. Of course, you have an instructor present to oversee what you are doing but I will never in my whole life forget walking into the nursing home, which was a nice new place, and immediately hearing a patient crying out, yelling and crying in misery. Back then, it was still legal to restrain a patient to "keep them safe" whatever that meant... I went into the facility and heard this poor woman who was sitting in what is called a geri chair and she was restrained with a posey vest, which tied her to that chair. The poor lady was not completely within her sound mind of course but it was very clear, she was absolutely miserable, she spent the entire time I was in that building crying and crying and crying and it was chilling.

I spent the entire semester in that nursing home for clinical rotation and that poor lady spent every day all day doing nothing but crying and sobbing and yelling, it was the most terrible thing I had ever seen. I remember asking if she ever had family visit her and they said no. My god, can you imagine being that poor woman?

That is exactly what the problem is. No one puts themselves in the patient's place. Not really, not good enough. I can honestly say I would rather die than live like that suffering all day and night every day, being tied down everywhere so I didn't wander off. My god. There are some things I just don't understand why they have to ever happen to anyone ever. That is one of them.

It was not too many years later that restraints were outlawed and now they are not used. The new saying was a patient has a right to fall. Isn't that weird? Restraints were outlawed because there were patients who were found dead in their hospital beds, in their geri chairs or wherever they were being used and the patients would attempt to get up out of bed and since most of them were not being checked on as often as they should have, they would get caught in between the hospital bed and the restraint and hang themselves or hang themselves from the restraints accidentally in other ways also. So very tragic, they finally outlawed them.

I have said to everyone who knows me that when I am old if for some tragic reason I have no one and my children dare put me in a nursing home, when I die, I will haunt them. I know that is not very nice to say but if they know how I feel about nursing homes and why I feel that way, they do not care about me one bit if they put me there because they don't want to take care of me. I would not put my worst enemy in a nursing home. Only criminals who have engaged in heinous crimes against other people belong in there. Now, I have said how I feel about them, I will move on.

There are now other alternatives to the standard process and levels of care a person can be referred to; there are assisted living facilities, group homes and live in help. I didn't really elaborate on those because they are expensive. Insurance does not cover them unless you have long-term care insurance. If you do, you are very lucky because they will also pay for equipment Medicare does not pay for and will even pay for PCA services at home, even if you do have family who is willing to help you.

Assisted Living Facilities in Las Vegas, Nevada range from $3000.00 a month to $10,000.00 a month. There are not many people who can afford that. They are usually very luxurious and the patient must be able to function pretty well on their own but may just need medication administration because they forget to take it or meal preparation because they left the stove on and almost burned the house down, maybe they need transportation to shopping and cannot drive and their families live in another state. There are many reasons for living in assisted living facilities. I have been a sub-contracted assessment nurse for a couple of friends who own a PCA service who does not accept Medicaid. They only service patients who have long term care insurance or can afford to pay cash. Long term insurance companies sometimes need nurses to assess the patient to see how much assistance the patient needs so they know how much help to allow the patient to have and be covered under their policy, sometimes they are patients who live in assisted living facilities and I go to assess them. I think most of the assisted living facilities I have visited are pretty good. Most of the patients I have met are fairly happy there. Sometimes they may not like it if it is a new experience because their caregiver/spouse passed away and they miss them, but for the most part, I have not had a real bad feeling about them, only that they are way too expensive.

Group homes are questionable; for the most part I definitely do not like them. I am not as bothered about them as I am nursing homes, but I would not want to stay in one and most of the patients I have seen there are not happy.

There are memory care facilities for people who are affected by dementia to the point they are no longer safe and may wander if not supervised 24/7 in a locked memory care facility. Those are very expensive and are usually very nice. The staff was always helpful there and for the most part, as far as I could tell, people appeared to be fairly happy. It is very difficult to judge happiness of a person with no memory. I never saw anything disturbing when I was in a memory care facility doing an assessment though. The diagnosis alone, however, is very tragic to me.

So, now that we have discussed places one may be discharged, what do we do if we are not ready to go home and have no help but don't want to be sent to skilled nursing or a nursing home? I will discuss that in the next chapter about appeals.

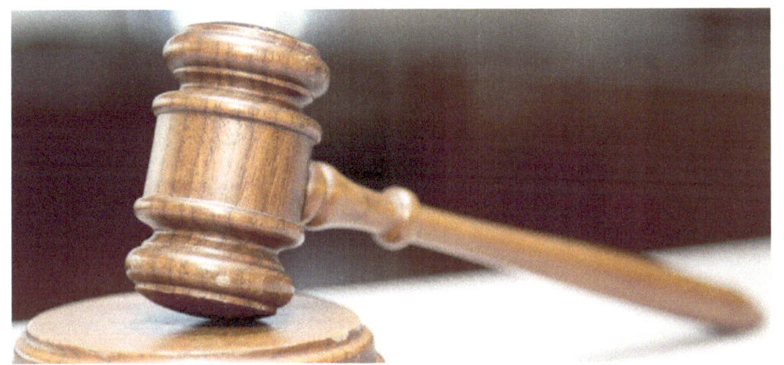

CHAPTER EIGHT
APPEAL RIGHTS

A lot of people are unaware that if you are a patient in the hospital and a case manager or a nurse tells you it is time to go home and they say you will be discharged that day or the next day and this is the first you may have heard about it or maybe you already have been told and are aware of the plan to discharge you that day or the next or whatever the case may be, you do not have to leave the hospital. Yep, I said, you do not have to leave. You have a right to tell your case manager or your nurse in the hospital that you want to appeal the decision to send you home. Just tell them that you are not feeling comfortable to go home yet and you think you are being discharged too soon.

In the hospital, every patient is supposed to be given what is called a NOMNC (Notice Of Medicare Non-Coverage). That paper gives you the information you need to start your appeal. You call the 800 number on the paper and inform the person who answers that you are a patient in the hospital and the hospital is attempting to discharge you home and you are not comfortable with that and you wish to appeal. At that point, the person on the line will gather your information and then call the facility and request your entire chart be sent to the insurance company/Medicare or whoever your insurer is, and the people who are in charge of appeals will review the entire chart and determine if you should be able to continue your hospitalization or if it is time to be discharged.

The review must also include a physician. There is a physician who will review your chart and may request to speak to your physician in the hospital to help make the determination.

What a lot of people don't know is, when a person requests an appeal, they automatically get two extra days in the hospital. That just happens automatically, even if the determination is that you should be discharged, there is no charge to the patient for staying the extra two days. The extra two days can actually make a big difference in a person's readiness to go home. It may give the physical therapy team that extra time needed to get you comfortable with being discharged. Sometimes even if the experts feel you are strong enough, you may still be afraid you aren't this may give you more time to feel more confident.

This is available to every patient in a hospital. Every patient is supposed to be informed of this but sometimes the case manager or nurse may not explain it well enough for you to fully understand exactly what it means.

If you feel worried about leaving the hospital because you feel you are not ready, PLEASE REQUEST AN APPEAL. IT IS YOUR RIGHT AS A PATIENT.

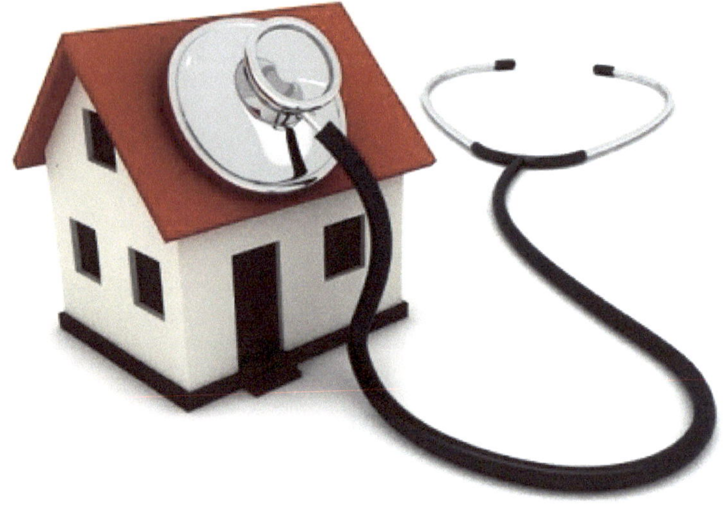

Most of the time when a patient is discharged home from the hospital, whether it is an acute care facility or a Skilled Nursing Facility, the physician will usually order home health care for you. Home Health Care is something every patient should take advantage of when it is offered to them. It is covered by your insurance company, no matter who that is. Medicare or any private insurer will pay for home health care when a patient is discharged home from a hospital stay.

It is the job of the home health company to transition you safely back to your environment after the misfortune of being in the hospital.

The case manager at the hospital is the person who is responsible to set it up once they receive the order from the physician. Sometimes the physician will specify what type of home health services are needed in their orders and sometimes they just order home health. When basic orders are received by the home health company, the scheduler will contact one of the Registered Nurses employed by their company to see if they can visit the patient within 48 hours maximum after discharge. If the nurse accepts the patient, they have 48 hours from discharge from the hospital to do the initial assessment to determine what services the patient will need. It is up to the Registered Nurse to evaluate the patient and order the appropriate disciplines to visit the patient. The home health registered nurse becomes the new case manager and is the "leader" of your team.

The registered nurse is usually able to decide if the patient should have a nurse visit them between 1-3 times per week at first to closely monitor your condition and watch for signs/symptoms that you need to go back to the hospital or be seen immediately by the physician for. It is their goal to keep you out of the hospital after you are discharged.

There are exceptions to that frequency; there may be a need for the nurse to see you every day at home and actually, sometimes more than once a day. Sometimes you will need IV antibiotics and it is best to get them from home if they will be needed long-term (commonly 6 weeks). It would be dreadful to have to be in the hospital for that reason alone and it is cheaper for your insurance company to pay for a nurse to come to your house daily than to pay for you to stay in the hospital anyway.

If you are discharged home with a terrible wound that requires daily dressing changes and you are unable to change the dressing yourself, the nurse may come daily for that reason. Sometimes you may have a wound which requires a wound vac which needs to be changed every 3 days or more frequently if there are complications.

If either of those situations occurs, however, there will always be a need for a family member or caregiver to be willing to be taught how to either administer your IV antibiotics through a long-term IV line that must be maintained very diligently or must be taught how to change your dressing; the exception would be the wound vac scenario. That is the only time the nurse would continue to come regularly sometimes for weeks, depending on how long it takes for the wound vac to no longer be needed.

There is also one other situation that is somewhat new. Most home health nurses have never managed this but it is called a pleural drain. It is placed into the peritoneal cavity and exits your body between your ribs on your side about midway of the torso, it requires draining of fluid that if not drained will definitely cause you to have difficulty breathing and will require hospital visits to have it drained in a more uncomfortable manner. The drain is a tube approximately 3cm in diameter and has a connector on the end which closes it off while it is not accessed by a special drainage canister set that will be sent to your house prior to the nurse coming to your house. There is also another kit for the dressing change, after the draining is completed, this holds the tube in place to keep it from dislodging /moving around, which would then cause discomfort, render the drain unusable and require a visit to the emergency room to have it replaced.

The pleural drain is also sutured to the skin to attempt to stabilize its position as well; however, after accessing it every 2- 3 days, it is common that the sutures may fall off. The nurse will take great care removing the dressing from the site, so as to not dislodge the drain, the nurse will then clean the connector with alcohol wipe that is in the kit, then attach the drain and a clear-straw colored fluid will fill the bag or bottle (depending on the brand of drain you have). The amount of drainage can vary greatly. In my experience, it will usually be between 100 ml and 1500ml with each draining. The fluid should appear a clear straw color, however, it may be red with blood, but still clear as it should be diluted by the fluid and not pure blood, or it may be an amber color, which is also indicative of blood but may also be cloudy if there is any puss. That is why the registered nurse should be the only person draining your drain, so they are frequently assessing the amount and the appearance of the drainage and will know when it is necessary for you to immediately seek the attention of a physician.

After the drainage is complete, the nurse will discard the fluid in a red biohazard bag and apply sterile gloves and perform sterile dressing placement, this will require cleansing the connector with alcohol, changing the clamp with the new one provided in the kit and coiling the drain tube, using steri-strips to secure it to the patient's side and cover with the provided sterile gauze and then placing a clear tegaderm dressing on top of that which is rather large and awkward but will help hold the dressing and tubing in place to protect the integrity of the drain. If the physician does not specify how often to do this, it will be up to the registered nurse's discretion and that should be determined by having a conversation with the patient to determine how long it takes between visits for the patient to feel like they are becoming short of breath with minimal activity, if the patient is unaware, it would just be based on how much drainage the nurse is getting when they drain the drain. So, there is some room to modify according to the patient's needs if the exact instructions are not written in the order by the physician. It is my opinion that it would be best for the nurse to have the ability to determine the frequency.

If a patient has suffered a fracture and required surgery to fix it, the patient will likely need physical and/or occupational therapy. Physical therapy is mainly focusing on your mobility; being safe to walk around or transfer to and from bed and the toilet. Occupational therapy is focusing on being able to feed yourself, helping you obtain adaptive equipment if you need it, helping you safely shower and getting things like reachers and grabbers. Most people don't know what Occupational therapy is and they think it has to do with working; it is actually focusing on fine motor skills.

When a patient suffers a brain injury, whether traumatic or a stroke or aneurysm, sometimes they are unable to speak without slurring and may be unable to find their words at all. This is very frustrating and will require the expertise of a speech /language pathologist. Home Health companies should also have access to Speech therapists they can send to evaluate you if it is something that is needed.

There are also nutritionists if a patient needs a tube feeding or having failure to thrive problems. These are rarely available in home health settings; however, some companies do have access to them and will send one to evaluate you if necessary.

All of the above therapy disciplines will do their own assessments and determine their frequencies according to their assessments of your needs.

Nursing will be determined by the Registered Nurse, the LPN and the CNA must be supervised by the Registered Nurse and will follow the frequency determined by the Registered Nurse at the initial assessment. The Registered Nurse is required to perform supervisory visits if you are being seen by a LPN or if you have CNA services once per month for LPN supervision and once every 2 weeks for CNA supervision.

Depending on the reason a patient is hospitalized will usually determine how long home healthcare is needed. You will be re-evaluated by the Registered Nurse after 9 weeks to see if you are ready for safe discharge, if so, you will be discharged, if not you may be recertified. If you are recertified, it will be for another 9-week period.

A patient should be discharged from home healthcare when they are safe to be discharged from home healthcare and skilled services are no longer needed, whether they are in the middle of a certification period, at the end of a certification period or at the beginning of a certification period, that should never make any difference. The most important indicator should be when the patient is ready to be safely discharged. That decision is usually up to the home health Registered Nurse. That decision is actually up to the physician. The home health company is not allowed to see the patient unless there is a physician's order.

Every time there is a change or new certification period, the new careplan must be sent to the primary care physician for approval and they must sign the careplan. The careplan is determined by the Registered Nurse or the Director of Nursing at the home health agency. Once it is signed, it serves at the physician's order for the certification period. A care plan states the problems the patient has, what the nurse plans to do about them (goals) and the interventions the nurse plans to use to reach those goals. The ultimate goal is to teach the patient how to safely deal with the problems they had when in the hospital if they have chronic effects and how to remain safe at home and stay out of the hospital.

I am sure it would be no surprise to anyone to learn I have spent several years of my nursing career being the Director of Nursing for home health agencies.   We all know by now how much I do not like hospitals.

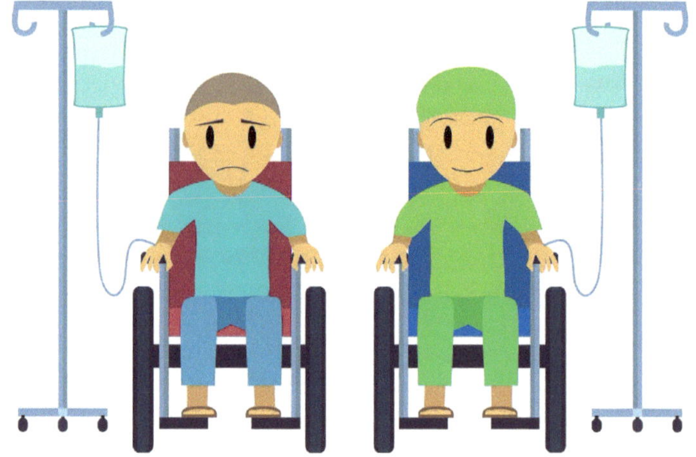

I have spent a lot of time throughout this book telling you everything that is bad about hospitals, doctors and nurses, however, it is very important to understand why. I am doing this to help you stay alive, to hopefully avoid anyone who may take the time to read this from having these terrible things happen to them. That is very important to me. That being said, I should also tell you….be a good patient, remember that you are not the only patient these professionals, who are there to help you, are taking care of. Try to understand that your nurse has a lot of medication to give to people and needs to be able to do it carefully and pay close attention to those five rights I told you about earlier.

I have never before seen such an amazing display of being a good patient in my life as I did when my mother was a patient in the hospital and was there for an extended period of time after I found her on the floor twice having a feeling of impending doom, later discovering she had 4 of 5 coronary arteries blocked (85%, 90%, 95% and 98%) and she had a severely stenotic aortic valve (opening only about 10%).

When my mother was in the hospital, she endured getting stuck every 3 days to have new peripheral IV sites placed (they are only good for 3 days), multiple lab draws to test her blood and monitor it very closely, she had a huge IV placed in her neck that had a pacemaker in it to help her heart after the valve replacement and an incision in her wrist. After she was sent home from that, she went back about 10 days later and had 2 stents placed and had an incision in her groin along with a couple of peripheral IV sticks.

My mother did not complain one time, never did she say she was afraid, she never complained that anything hurt, she never was ever in a grouchy mood, she was so sweet to everyone who came in her room for any reason and thanked them for everything every single time, even if it was something that hurt. I have never in my life seen anything like it. I was in awe. All the nurses and doctors loved her, after her surgery for the valve replacement, the anesthesiologist ran to me and told me he loved my mother and asked if she could adopt him and said he wanted to come to our house for dinner. It was the most amazing thing I had ever seen.

When she went back to have her stents placed, she was in the operating room, having the procedure done and a song came on that she liked overhead and she said "Oh, I like that song"! My mother said that while she was underneath the drape and the doctor was actually doing the procedure. She said everyone laughed when she said that. I can imagine so, who does that? Most people are scared, in a bad mood and could care less what song is playing in the operating room when they are being worked on.

There are 2 benefits to this behavior as a patient; not only will your chances be much greater of a fast and positive recovery, but, everyone who you come in contact with will love you for being so pleasant and will likely be nicer to you and want to do more to help you, unfortunately it will matter like that. People should want to help you anyway but I guarantee; people will be more likely to help you and be nice if you are nice and pleasant to them and don't act like you are the only patient they are taking care of.

I myself don't even know if I would be able to be as amazing as my mother through something like she experienced but I can only pray I will. It was a definite eye opener and I learned so much about what a difference a patient's attitude has on their illness/ recovery/ the way they will ultimately be treated by everyone they encounter and I have the utmost respect for my mother's example of soldier-like bravery in the situation she was in.

Only 2 weeks after being discharged from the hospital, my mother was moving across the country to Texas by herself to be near her boyfriend as is having the time of her life. Yes, I miss her greatly, but she is happy, so I am happy for her.

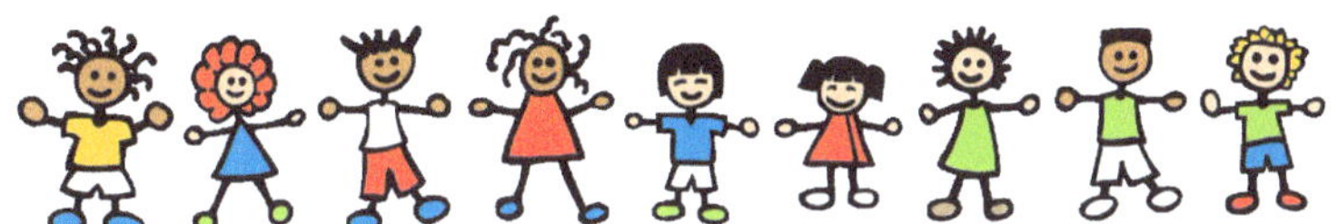

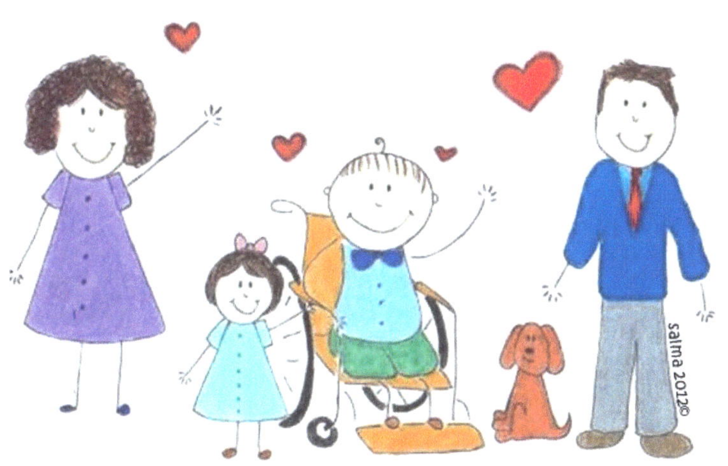

CHAPTER ELEVEN
FAMILY

One thing I feel is necessary to discuss is family. You are the patient, you don't feel good, yes, that is very true. Please do not forget that your family/loved ones are also experiencing a very frightening time when they are worried about what has just happened to you. They are scared, don't know what to do to help and also, likely, have lives of their own. Many of them likely have jobs that they still have to attend every day. It is hard for them to be able to continue their normal routine and then go to the hospital after work to help make sure everything is going smoothly with your care. Family members often become exhausted.

The old saying is sometimes true; we are sometimes harder on the people we love the most, we can at times be too expecting of these people, expect them to be super human and even get appalled that they act like they are so bothered, thinking, "I am the one who is sick, what are they complaining about?" Is that really fair? No! Who do they have to talk to about their feelings, their fears about what is happening to their loved one? No one a lot of times. Try also putting yourself in their shoes and think if it was them in the hospital, how worried you would likely be and if you had to add all of that to your daily routine, how exhausted you would likely be.

Remember how lucky you are to have someone who cares enough about you to even come visit at all or ask what is happening. It is very sad how many people do not have that.

Don't take that for granted, don't be mean to them, they are there because they care about you, appreciate that and treat them like you would want to be treated if that was you.

Be sure to get your family involved in your care. It is important for your safety and people will be more careful how they treat you if they know there is someone watching out for you, it is sad, but true.

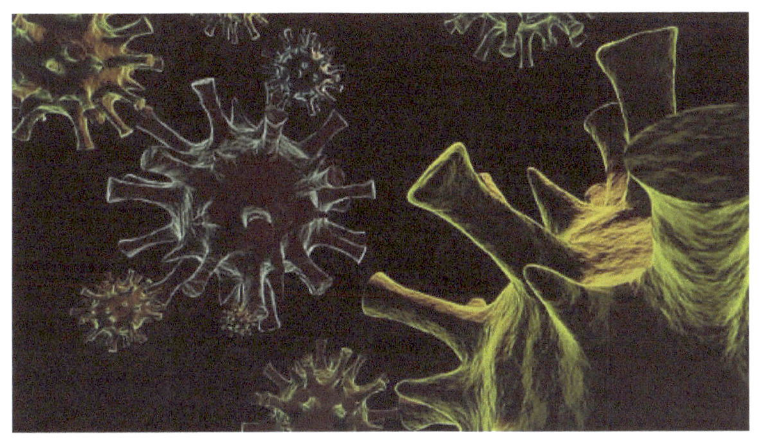

CHAPTER TWELVE
THE CONSIDERATIONS REGARDING COVID-19

Unfortunately, since the onset of COVID-19, there have been many changes and uncertainties. I am going to give my advice in this chapter, it is only based on the knowledge I have gained to date from many different settings; meetings with other healthcare professionals, news casts I have seen and common sense conclusions I have drawn based on the information I have obtained.

It is my opinion as a Registered Nurse of 20 years that there is still not enough known about COVID-19. I am making this statement on July 1, 2020. Since this began, there have been varying statements of how long the virus stays alive on surfaces of varying materials and in the air and so forth, I am a firm believer in err on the cautious side, everyone wear masks please, wear them as instructed as they are meant to be worn. I see so many people wearing masks underneath their exposed nose. Really? That is not doing any good! Wear them over the nose mouth and chin and crimp the nose clip to fit your face for god's sake.

People have a tendency to become desensitized. It seems to be human nature or something, if you think about it, just think about it, when you hear about something scary or terrible, it is shocking and it frightens you, right? Well, after a few days or however long, the next time you hear about it, it loses its shock factor, you have heard it before, so you aren't as surprised about the contents. If you don't have it in your face every minute, you go on throughout the day and about your life and get back to being caught-up in your daily routine, in the problems that are effecting you already that you are already dealing with and that is your immediate focus. Suddenly, it just seems to be that the horrible and scary thing you heard about is the last thing on your mind and if you continue to hear about it, whether it be updates or the same information over and over on the news, maybe even conflicting opinions about what to do about it or what it all means, it just seems to get lost in the shuffle of day-to-day life.

That is very scary. Especially when we are talking about a virus that is 6 times more infectious than influenza and is so brutal and is taking so many lives. We don't have a vaccine people! What is wrong with everyone? It is still the same horrible, scary virus it was the first time you heard about it…without a vaccine, nothing has changed, don't you understand that?

Taking temperatures of people who are going into a workplace or public place really does nothing. Most people with temperature feel horrible; they are probably the people at home or in the hospital. You can be a carrier and not have signs and symptoms, so just because you have no fever, you can go to work and into public places like everyone else and spread that terrible virus everywhere. It makes no sense to me.

Wear masks the right way, wear gloves when you are going to be touching anything someone who doesn't live with you has been touching (gas pumps, counters at stores), wipe off everything you get from the store with disinfectant before you bring it in your house, the virus lives on surfaces for days remember? Do this every time. Don't get lazy; your life depends on it. Stay home! Don't be in a crowd!

Don't get me wrong, I understand people have got to eat and have a place to live, I understand our country will be in a terrible mess with everything shut down but I don't understand people who do not follow the basic recommendations by the CDC, I said the CDC, they are the experts in disease control. HELLO!! They are not making recommendations to hear themselves speak, to feel important or to apply to everyone but you, they are telling everyone what to do to **try** to stay safe. They are giving advice on the best possible ways to stay safe that they have discovered based on scientific fact or experience by experts in the field of disease control. Since when did their advice mean nothing???

I am horrified at the lack of understanding that this advice comes from experts who spend their lives studying disease control and doing experiments and they are the only people to listen to.

In the medical profession, a physician is considered an expert in a court of law if they are testifying about something related to their field, a nurse is an expert in a court of law if they are testifying about something related to their field...expert means expert. It takes many years of education and experience to become an expert in something so filled with responsibility for human lives...do you get what I am saying? Listen to the CDC, do what they recommend, don't put your life at risk and if you don't care about your own life, please be considerate enough to care about putting other lives at risk and follow the recommendations!! This virus is no joke.

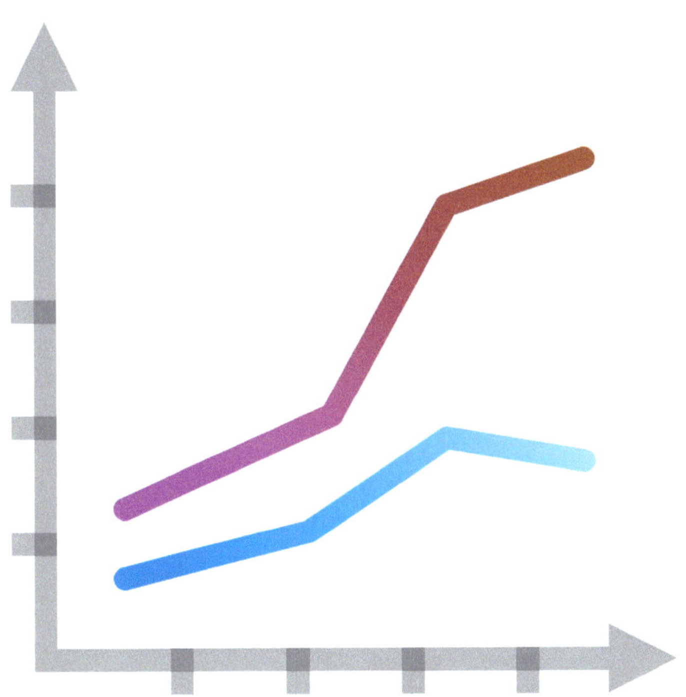

I did some research to let you know about some very important statistics I think everyone should know.

The first category, Adverse Events; these are Adverse drug events, Healthcare Acquired Infections (HCAIs) and Surgical complications.

1.7 Million Patients annually acquire HCAIs while being treated for other health issues.

98,000 patients (1 in 17) die due to HCAIs every year.

HCAIs are now killing more people than Cancer, HIV/AIDS or road traffic accidents.

A survey conducted in 183 US hospitals with 11,282 patients reported 4% had at least one HCAI, most commonly Clostridium Difficile. Most infections were surgical site infections, pneumonia and gastrointestinal infections.

Although the statistics I gave you represent the United States, they are also problematic in other countries.

"Never Events" - There is a list of Never Events that are mistakes made in the field of medical treatment. See below:

1. Artificial insemination with the wrong donor sperm or egg.
2. Unintended retention of a foreign body in a patient after surgery or other procedure.
3. Patient death or serious disability associated with patient elopement (disappearance).
4. Patient death or serious disability associated with a medication error.
5. Patient death or serious disability associated with a hemolytic reaction due to the administration of ABO/HLA-incompatible blood or blood products.
6. Patient death or serious disability associated with an electric shock or elective cardioversion while being cared for in a healthcare facility.

7. Patient death or serious disability associated with a fall while being cared for in a healthcare facility.
8. Surgery performed on the wrong body part.
9. Surgery performed on the wrong patient.
10. Wrong surgical procedure performed on a patient.
11. Intraoperative or immediately postoperative death in an ASA Class I patient.
12. Patient death or serious disability associated with the use of contaminated drugs, devices, or biologics provided by the healthcare facility.
13. Patient death or serious disability associated with the use or function of a device in patient care, in which the device is used or functions other as intended.
14. Patient death or serious disability associated with intravascular air embolism that occurs while being cared for in a healthcare facility.
15. Infant discharged to the wrong person.
16. Patient suicide, or attempted suicide resulting in serious disability, while being cared for in a healthcare facility,
17. Maternal death or serious disability associated with labor or delivery in a low-risk pregnancy while being cared for in a healthcare facility.
18. Patient death or serious disability associated with hypoglycemia, the onset which occurs while the patient is being cared for in a health care facility.
19. Death or serious disability (kernicterus) associated with failure to identify and treat hyperbilirubinemia in neonates.
20. Stage 3 or 4 pressure ulcers acquired after admission to a healthcare facility.
21. Patient death or serious disability due to spinal manipulative therapy.
22. Any incident in which a line designated for oxygen or other gas to be delivered to a patient contains the wrong gas or is contaminated by toxic substances.
23. Patient death or serious disability associated with a burn incurred from any source while being cared for in a healthcare facility.

24. Patient death or serious disability associated with the use of restraints or bedrails while being cared for in a healthcare facility.
25. Any instance of care ordered by or provided by someone impersonating a physician, nurse, pharmacist or other licensed healthcare provider.
26. Abduction of a patient of any age.
27. Sexual assault on a patient within or on the grounds of the healthcare facility.
28. Death or significant injury of a patient or staff member resulting from a physical assault that occurs within or on the grounds of the healthcare facility.

It is estimated 33,000 plus lives could be saved if all hospitals performed at the level of those hospitals which received "A" grade from The Leapfrog Group.

The Leapfrog Group, founded in 2000 by large employers and other purchasers, The Leapfrog Group is a national nonprofit organization driving a movement for giant leaps forward in the quality and safety of American health care. The flagship Leapfrog Hospital Survey collects and transparently reports hospital performance, empowering purchasers to find the highest-value care and giving consumers the life-saving information they need to make informed decisions. The Leapfrog Hospital Safety Grade, Leapfrog's other main initiative; assigns letter grades to hospitals based on their record of patient safety, helping consumers protect themselves and their families from errors, injuries, accidents, and infections.

Each year, Adverse Drug Events account for nearly 700,000 Emergency Room visits and 100,000 hospitalizations.

Nearly 5% of hospitalized patients experience an ADE making them one of the most common types of inpatient errors.

Then there are the readmissions to the hospitals within 30 days of discharge:

There are over 35 million hospital discharges annually in the United States.

The cost of unplanned readmissions is 15-20 billion dollars annually.

13-17% of Medicare patients discharged from hospitals is readmitted within 30 days.

U.S. physicians say up to 30% of medical services are unnecessary.

The top 3 reasons physicians cited for over treatment was fear of malpractice (84.7%), pressure from patients (59%) and difficulty accessing prior medical record of patients (38.2%). Other reasons cited included inadequate time spent with patients, pressure from colleagues and medical institutions or management, as well as concerns about "looking good" in performance evaluations.

And finally, the frightening reality of healthcare workers practicing while impaired. It is estimated that approximately 15% of physicians practice while impaired and 10-15% of nurses practice while impaired.

REFERENCES

1. Collins AS. Preventing Health Care-Associated Infections. In: Hughes RG, editor. Patient Safety and Quality: An Evidence-Based Handbook for Nurses. Rockville (MD): Agency for Healthcare Research and Quality (US); 2008. Apr, [Accessed June 30, 2020]. Chapter 41. Available from: https://www.ncbi.nlm.nih.gov/books/NBK2683/ [Google Scholar]
2. Resnick, Richard. "There's Much Work to Be Done: 8 Medical Errors Statistics to Know." *cureatr*(blog), February 19, 2019, [Accessed June 30, 2020] Available from: https://blog.cureatr.com/theres-much-work-to-be-done-8-medical-errors-statistics-to-know
3. "Never Event", Wikipedia, Wikimedia Foundation, May 25, 2020, [Accessed June 30, 2020]. Available from: https://en.wikipedia.org/wiki/Never_event
4. "Medication Errors and Adverse Drug Events" , PSNet, September 2019, [Accessed June 30, 2020] Available from: https://psnet.ahrq.gov/primer/medication-errors-and-adverse-drug-events

5. Alper, Eric, MD, O'Malley, Terrence A., MD, Greenwald, Jeffrey, MD, "Hospital Discharge and Readmission", UpToDate, June 2020, [Accessed June 30, 2020] Available from: https://www.uptodate.com/contents/hospital-discharge-and-readmission

6. Perry, Susan, "U.S. Physicians Say Up to 30 Percent of Medical Services are Unnecessary" MINNPOST, September 12, 2017, [Accessed June 30, 2020] Available from: https://www.minnpost.com/second-opinion/2017/09/us-physicians-say-30-percent-medical-services-are-unnecessary/

7. Lockhart, Lisa, MHA, MSN, RN, NE-BC, Davis, Charlotte, BSN, RN, CCRN "Spotting Imapairment in the Healthcare Workplace", Lippincott Nursing Center, [Accessed June 30, 2020] Available from: https://www.nursingcenter.com/ce_articleprint?an=00152258-201705000-00009

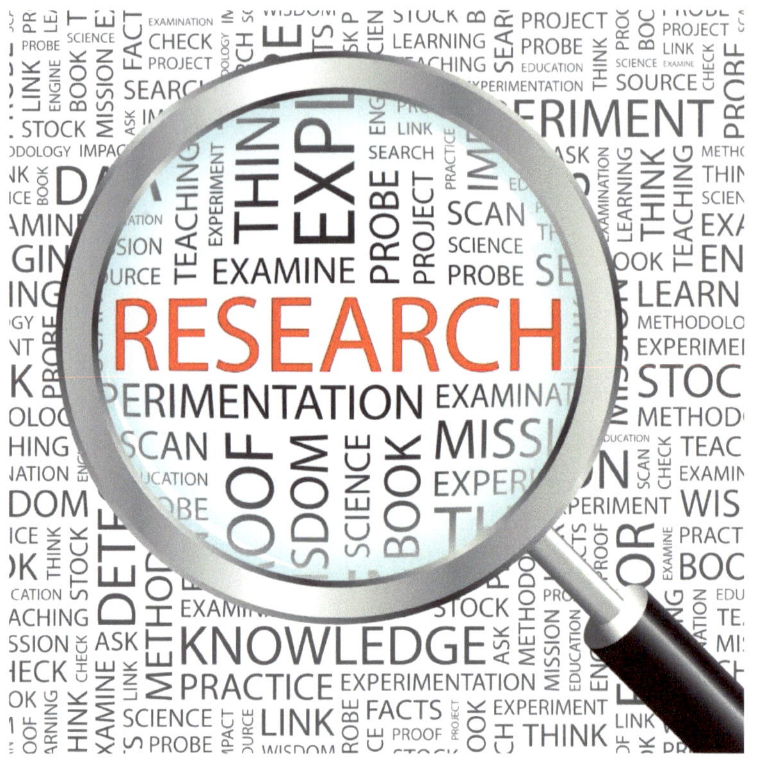

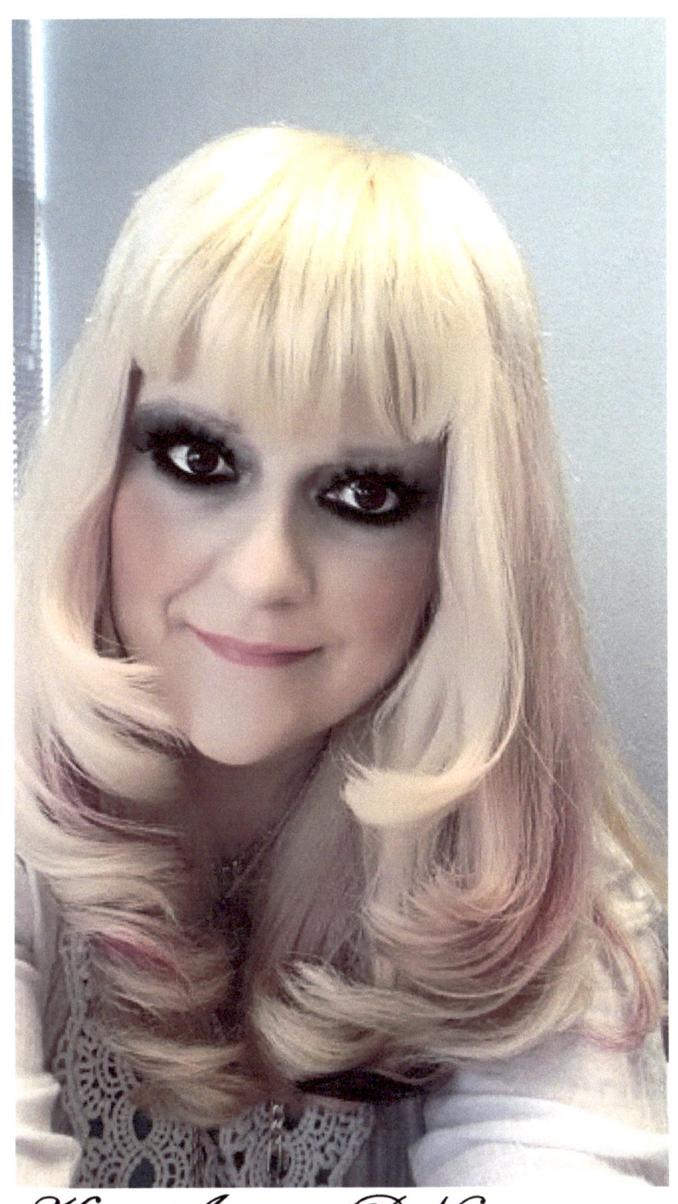

Kristy Anderson RN